THE FAT TO FIT LOG

NAME:

AGE:

CURRENT WEIGHT:

TARGETED WEIGHT:

LOG COMPLETE WEIGHT:

DATE/DAY:			M	T	W	T	F	S	S
START TIME:		FINISH TIME:							

CARDIO TRAINING

TRAINING TYPE	TARGETED TIME /DISTANCE	ACTUAL TIME /DISTANCE	CALORIES BURNED

STRENGTH TRAINING

TRAINING TYPE	TARGETED MUSCLE GROUP		SETS					
-----	-----		1	2	3	4	5	6
		REPS						
		WGT						
		REPS						
		WGT						
		REPS						
		WGT						
		REPS						
		WGT						
		REPS						
		WGT						
		REPS						
		WGT						
		REPS						
		WGT						

REFLECTION OF THE DAY

DATE/DAY:			M	T	W	T	F	S	S
START TIME:		FINISH TIME:							

CARDIO TRAINING

TRAINING TYPE	TARGETED TIME /DISTANCE	ACTUAL TIME /DISTANCE	CALORIES BURNED

STRENGTH TRAINING

TRAINING TYPE	TARGETED MUSCLE GROUP		SETS					
-----	-----		**1**	**2**	**3**	**4**	**5**	**6**
		REPS						
		WGT						
		REPS						
		WGT						
		REPS						
		WGT						
		REPS						
		WGT						
		REPS						
		WGT						
		REPS						
		WGT						
		REPS						
		WGT						

REFLECTION OF THE DAY

DATE/DAY:				M	T	W	T	F	S	S
START TIME:		FINISH TIME:								

CARDIO TRAINING

TRAINING TYPE	TARGETED TIME /DISTANCE	ACTUAL TIME /DISTANCE	CALORIES BURNED

STRENGTH TRAINING

TRAINING TYPE	TARGETED MUSCLE GROUP	SETS		1	2	3	4	5	6
-----	-----								
		REPS							
		WGT							
		REPS							
		WGT							
		REPS							
		WGT							
		REPS							
		WGT							
		REPS							
		WGT							
		REPS							
		WGT							
		REPS							
		WGT							

REFLECTION OF THE DAY

DATE/DAY:				M	T	W	T	F	S	S
START TIME:		FINISH TIME:								

CARDIO TRAINING

TRAINING TYPE	TARGETED TIME /DISTANCE	ACTUAL TIME /DISTANCE	CALORIES BURNED

STRENGTH TRAINING

TRAINING TYPE	TARGETED MUSCLE GROUP		SETS					
-----	-----		**1**	**2**	**3**	**4**	**5**	**6**
		REPS						
		WGT						
		REPS						
		WGT						
		REPS						
		WGT						
		REPS						
		WGT						
		REPS						
		WGT						
		REPS						
		WGT						
		REPS						
		WGT						

REFLECTION OF THE DAY

DATE/DAY:		M	T	W	T	F	S	S
START TIME:	FINISH TIME:							

CARDIO TRAINING

TRAINING TYPE	TARGETED TIME /DISTANCE	ACTUAL TIME /DISTANCE	CALORIES BURNED

STRENGTH TRAINING

TRAINING TYPE	TARGETED MUSCLE GROUP		SETS					
-----	-----		**1**	**2**	**3**	**4**	**5**	**6**
		REPS						
		WGT						
		REPS						
		WGT						
		REPS						
		WGT						
		REPS						
		WGT						
		REPS						
		WGT						
		REPS						
		WGT						
		REPS						
		WGT						

REFLECTION OF THE DAY

DATE/DAY:				M	T	W	T	F	S	S
START TIME:		FINISH TIME:								

CARDIO TRAINING

TRAINING TYPE	TARGETED TIME /DISTANCE	ACTUAL TIME /DISTANCE	CALORIES BURNED

STRENGTH TRAINING

TRAINING TYPE	TARGETED MUSCLE GROUP	SETS	1	2	3	4	5	6
-----	-----							
		REPS						
		WGT						
		REPS						
		WGT						
		REPS						
		WGT						
		REPS						
		WGT						
		REPS						
		WGT						
		REPS						
		WGT						
		REPS						
		WGT						

REFLECTION OF THE DAY

DATE/DAY:		M	T	W	T	F	S	S
START TIME:		FINISH TIME:						

CARDIO TRAINING

TRAINING TYPE	TARGETED TIME /DISTANCE	ACTUAL TIME /DISTANCE	CALORIES BURNED

STRENGTH TRAINING

TRAINING TYPE	TARGETED MUSCLE GROUP		SETS					
-----	-----		**1**	**2**	**3**	**4**	**5**	**6**
		REPS						
		WGT						
		REPS						
		WGT						
		REPS						
		WGT						
		REPS						
		WGT						
		REPS						
		WGT						
		REPS						
		WGT						
		REPS						
		WGT						

REFLECTION OF THE DAY

<table>
<tr><td>DATE/DAY:</td><td></td><td>M</td><td>T</td><td>W</td><td>T</td><td>F</td><td>S</td><td>S</td></tr>
<tr><td>START TIME:</td><td colspan="2">FINISH TIME:</td><td colspan="6"></td></tr>
</table>

CARDIO TRAINING

TRAINING TYPE	TARGETED TIME /DISTANCE	ACTUAL TIME /DISTANCE	CALORIES BURNED

STRENGTH TRAINING

TRAINING TYPE	TARGETED MUSCLE GROUP	SETS		1	2	3	4	5	6
-----	-----								
		REPS							
		WGT							
		REPS							
		WGT							
		REPS							
		WGT							
		REPS							
		WGT							
		REPS							
		WGT							
		REPS							
		WGT							
		REPS							
		WGT							

REFLECTION OF THE DAY

| DATE/DAY: | | | M | T | W | T | F | S | S |
| START TIME: | | FINISH TIME: | | | | | | | |

CARDIO TRAINING

TRAINING TYPE	TARGETED TIME /DISTANCE	ACTUAL TIME /DISTANCE	CALORIES BURNED

STRENGTH TRAINING

TRAINING TYPE	TARGETED MUSCLE GROUP	SETS		1	2	3	4	5	6
-----	-----								
		REPS							
		WGT							
		REPS							
		WGT							
		REPS							
		WGT							
		REPS							
		WGT							
		REPS							
		WGT							
		REPS							
		WGT							
		REPS							
		WGT							

REFLECTION OF THE DAY

DATE/DAY:			M	T	W	T	F	S	S
START TIME:		FINISH TIME:							

CARDIO TRAINING

TRAINING TYPE	TARGETED TIME /DISTANCE	ACTUAL TIME /DISTANCE	CALORIES BURNED

STRENGTH TRAINING

TRAINING TYPE	TARGETED MUSCLE GROUP		SETS					
-----	-----		**1**	**2**	**3**	**4**	**5**	**6**
		REPS						
		WGT						
		REPS						
		WGT						
		REPS						
		WGT						
		REPS						
		WGT						
		REPS						
		WGT						
		REPS						
		WGT						
		REPS						
		WGT						

REFLECTION OF THE DAY

<table>
<tr><td>DATE/DAY:</td><td></td><td>M</td><td>T</td><td>W</td><td>T</td><td>F</td><td>S</td><td>S</td></tr>
<tr><td>START TIME:</td><td colspan="2">FINISH TIME:</td><td colspan="6"></td></tr>
</table>

CARDIO TRAINING

TRAINING TYPE	TARGETED TIME /DISTANCE	ACTUAL TIME /DISTANCE	CALORIES BURNED

STRENGTH TRAINING

TRAINING TYPE	TARGETED MUSCLE GROUP		SETS					
-----	-----		**1**	**2**	**3**	**4**	**5**	**6**
		REPS						
		WGT						
		REPS						
		WGT						
		REPS						
		WGT						
		REPS						
		WGT						
		REPS						
		WGT						
		REPS						
		WGT						
		REPS						
		WGT						

REFLECTION OF THE DAY

<table>
<tr><td colspan="2">DATE/DAY:</td><td>M</td><td>T</td><td>W</td><td>T</td><td>F</td><td>S</td><td>S</td></tr>
<tr><td>START TIME:</td><td colspan="8">FINISH TIME:</td></tr>
</table>

CARDIO TRAINING

TRAINING TYPE	TARGETED TIME /DISTANCE	ACTUAL TIME /DISTANCE	CALORIES BURNED

STRENGTH TRAINING

TRAINING TYPE	TARGETED MUSCLE GROUP		SETS					
-----	-----		**1**	**2**	**3**	**4**	**5**	**6**
		REPS						
		WGT						
		REPS						
		WGT						
		REPS						
		WGT						
		REPS						
		WGT						
		REPS						
		WGT						
		REPS						
		WGT						
		REPS						
		WGT						

REFLECTION OF THE DAY

DATE/DAY:			M	T	W	T	F	S	S
START TIME:		FINISH TIME:							

CARDIO TRAINING

TRAINING TYPE	TARGETED TIME /DISTANCE	ACTUAL TIME /DISTANCE	CALORIES BURNED

STRENGTH TRAINING

TRAINING TYPE	TARGETED MUSCLE GROUP		SETS					
-----	-----		**1**	**2**	**3**	**4**	**5**	**6**
		REPS						
		WGT						
		REPS						
		WGT						
		REPS						
		WGT						
		REPS						
		WGT						
		REPS						
		WGT						
		REPS						
		WGT						
		REPS						
		WGT						

REFLECTION OF THE DAY

DATE/DAY:			M	T	W	T	F	S	S
START TIME:		FINISH TIME:							

CARDIO TRAINING

TRAINING TYPE	TARGETED TIME /DISTANCE	ACTUAL TIME /DISTANCE	CALORIES BURNED

STRENGTH TRAINING

TRAINING TYPE	TARGETED MUSCLE GROUP		SETS					
-----	-----		1	2	3	4	5	6
		REPS						
		WGT						
		REPS						
		WGT						
		REPS						
		WGT						
		REPS						
		WGT						
		REPS						
		WGT						
		REPS						
		WGT						
		REPS						
		WGT						

REFLECTION OF THE DAY

DATE/DAY:			M	T	W	T	F	S	S
START TIME:		FINISH TIME:							

CARDIO TRAINING

TRAINING TYPE	TARGETED TIME /DISTANCE	ACTUAL TIME /DISTANCE	CALORIES BURNED

STRENGTH TRAINING

TRAINING TYPE	TARGETED MUSCLE GROUP	SETS		1	2	3	4	5	6
-----	-----								
		REPS							
		WGT							
		REPS							
		WGT							
		REPS							
		WGT							
		REPS							
		WGT							
		REPS							
		WGT							
		REPS							
		WGT							
		REPS							
		WGT							

REFLECTION OF THE DAY

<table>
<tr><td>DATE/DAY:</td><td></td><td>M</td><td>T</td><td>W</td><td>T</td><td>F</td><td>S</td><td>S</td></tr>
<tr><td>START TIME:</td><td colspan="2">FINISH TIME:</td><td colspan="6"></td></tr>
</table>

CARDIO TRAINING

TRAINING TYPE	TARGETED TIME /DISTANCE	ACTUAL TIME /DISTANCE	CALORIES BURNED

STRENGTH TRAINING

TRAINING TYPE	TARGETED MUSCLE GROUP	SETS	1	2	3	4	5	6
-----	-----							
		REPS						
		WGT						
		REPS						
		WGT						
		REPS						
		WGT						
		REPS						
		WGT						
		REPS						
		WGT						
		REPS						
		WGT						
		REPS						
		WGT						

REFLECTION OF THE DAY

DATE/DAY:		M	T	W	T	F	S	S
START TIME:		FINISH TIME:						

CARDIO TRAINING

TRAINING TYPE	TARGETED TIME /DISTANCE	ACTUAL TIME /DISTANCE	CALORIES BURNED

STRENGTH TRAINING

TRAINING TYPE	TARGETED MUSCLE GROUP		SETS					
-----	-----		**1**	**2**	**3**	**4**	**5**	**6**
		REPS						
		WGT						
		REPS						
		WGT						
		REPS						
		WGT						
		REPS						
		WGT						
		REPS						
		WGT						
		REPS						
		WGT						
		REPS						
		WGT						

REFLECTION OF THE DAY

<table>
<tr><td>DATE/DAY:</td><td colspan="2"></td><td>M</td><td>T</td><td>W</td><td>T</td><td>F</td><td>S</td><td>S</td></tr>
<tr><td>START TIME:</td><td>FINISH TIME:</td><td colspan="8"></td></tr>
</table>

CARDIO TRAINING

TRAINING TYPE	TARGETED TIME /DISTANCE	ACTUAL TIME /DISTANCE	CALORIES BURNED

STRENGTH TRAINING

TRAINING TYPE	TARGETED MUSCLE GROUP	SETS	1	2	3	4	5	6
-----	-----		__1__	__2__	__3__	__4__	__5__	__6__
		REPS						
		WGT						
		REPS						
		WGT						
		REPS						
		WGT						
		REPS						
		WGT						
		REPS						
		WGT						
		REPS						
		WGT						
		REPS						
		WGT						

REFLECTION OF THE DAY

DATE/DAY:		M	T	W	T	F	S	S
START TIME:		FINISH TIME:						

CARDIO TRAINING

TRAINING TYPE	TARGETED TIME /DISTANCE	ACTUAL TIME /DISTANCE	CALORIES BURNED

STRENGTH TRAINING

TRAINING TYPE	TARGETED MUSCLE GROUP		SETS					
------	------		1	2	3	4	5	6
		REPS						
		WGT						
		REPS						
		WGT						
		REPS						
		WGT						
		REPS						
		WGT						
		REPS						
		WGT						
		REPS						
		WGT						
		REPS						
		WGT						

REFLECTION OF THE DAY

DATE/DAY:				M	T	W	T	F	S	S
START TIME:		FINISH TIME:								

CARDIO TRAINING

TRAINING TYPE	TARGETED TIME /DISTANCE	ACTUAL TIME /DISTANCE	CALORIES BURNED

STRENGTH TRAINING

TRAINING TYPE	TARGETED MUSCLE GROUP	SETS							
-----	-----		**1**	**2**	**3**	**4**	**5**	**6**
		REPS							
		WGT							
		REPS							
		WGT							
		REPS							
		WGT							
		REPS							
		WGT							
		REPS							
		WGT							
		REPS							
		WGT							
		REPS							
		WGT							

REFLECTION OF THE DAY

<table>
<tr><td>DATE/DAY:</td><td colspan="2"></td><td>M</td><td>T</td><td>W</td><td>T</td><td>F</td><td>S</td><td>S</td></tr>
<tr><td>START TIME:</td><td></td><td>FINISH TIME:</td><td colspan="7"></td></tr>
</table>

CARDIO TRAINING

TRAINING TYPE	TARGETED TIME /DISTANCE	ACTUAL TIME /DISTANCE	CALORIES BURNED

STRENGTH TRAINING

TRAINING TYPE	TARGETED MUSCLE GROUP	SETS						
-----	-----		1	2	3	4	5	6
		REPS						
		WGT						
		REPS						
		WGT						
		REPS						
		WGT						
		REPS						
		WGT						
		REPS						
		WGT						
		REPS						
		WGT						
		REPS						
		WGT						

REFLECTION OF THE DAY

DATE/DAY:				M	T	W	T	F	S	S
START TIME:		FINISH TIME:								

CARDIO TRAINING

TRAINING TYPE	TARGETED TIME /DISTANCE	ACTUAL TIME /DISTANCE	CALORIES BURNED

STRENGTH TRAINING

TRAINING TYPE	TARGETED MUSCLE GROUP		SETS					
-----	-----		**1**	**2**	**3**	**4**	**5**	**6**
		REPS						
		WGT						
		REPS						
		WGT						
		REPS						
		WGT						
		REPS						
		WGT						
		REPS						
		WGT						
		REPS						
		WGT						
		REPS						
		WGT						

REFLECTION OF THE DAY

DATE/DAY:		M	T	W	T	F	S	S
START TIME:	FINISH TIME:							

CARDIO TRAINING

TRAINING TYPE	TARGETED TIME /DISTANCE	ACTUAL TIME /DISTANCE	CALORIES BURNED

STRENGTH TRAINING

TRAINING TYPE	TARGETED MUSCLE GROUP		SETS					
-----	-----		**1**	**2**	**3**	**4**	**5**	**6**
		REPS						
		WGT						
		REPS						
		WGT						
		REPS						
		WGT						
		REPS						
		WGT						
		REPS						
		WGT						
		REPS						
		WGT						
		REPS						
		WGT						

REFLECTION OF THE DAY

<table>
<tr><td>DATE/DAY:</td><td></td><td>M</td><td>T</td><td>W</td><td>T</td><td>F</td><td>S</td><td>S</td></tr>
<tr><td>START TIME:</td><td>FINISH TIME:</td><td colspan="7"></td></tr>
</table>

CARDIO TRAINING

TRAINING TYPE	TARGETED TIME /DISTANCE	ACTUAL TIME /DISTANCE	CALORIES BURNED

STRENGTH TRAINING

TRAINING TYPE	TARGETED MUSCLE GROUP		SETS					
-----	-----		**1**	**2**	**3**	**4**	**5**	**6**
		REPS						
		WGT						
		REPS						
		WGT						
		REPS						
		WGT						
		REPS						
		WGT						
		REPS						
		WGT						
		REPS						
		WGT						
		REPS						
		WGT						

REFLECTION OF THE DAY

<table>
<tr><td>DATE/DAY:</td><td></td><td>M</td><td>T</td><td>W</td><td>T</td><td>F</td><td>S</td><td>S</td></tr>
<tr><td>START TIME:</td><td>FINISH TIME:</td><td colspan="7"></td></tr>
</table>

CARDIO TRAINING

TRAINING TYPE	TARGETED TIME /DISTANCE	ACTUAL TIME /DISTANCE	CALORIES BURNED

STRENGTH TRAINING

TRAINING TYPE	TARGETED MUSCLE GROUP		SETS					
-----	-----		1	2	3	4	5	6
		REPS						
		WGT						
		REPS						
		WGT						
		REPS						
		WGT						
		REPS						
		WGT						
		REPS						
		WGT						
		REPS						
		WGT						
		REPS						
		WGT						

REFLECTION OF THE DAY

DATE/DAY:			M	T	W	T	F	S	S
START TIME:		FINISH TIME:							

CARDIO TRAINING

TRAINING TYPE	TARGETED TIME /DISTANCE	ACTUAL TIME /DISTANCE	CALORIES BURNED

STRENGTH TRAINING

TRAINING TYPE	TARGETED MUSCLE GROUP	SETS							
-----	-----		**1**	**2**	**3**	**4**	**5**	**6**	
		REPS							
		WGT							
		REPS							
		WGT							
		REPS							
		WGT							
		REPS							
		WGT							
		REPS							
		WGT							
		REPS							
		WGT							
		REPS							
		WGT							

REFLECTION OF THE DAY

<table>
<tr><td>DATE/DAY:</td><td></td><td colspan="2">M</td><td>T</td><td>W</td><td>T</td><td>F</td><td>S</td><td>S</td></tr>
<tr><td>START TIME:</td><td></td><td>FINISH TIME:</td><td colspan="7"></td></tr>
</table>

CARDIO TRAINING

TRAINING TYPE	TARGETED TIME /DISTANCE	ACTUAL TIME /DISTANCE	CALORIES BURNED

STRENGTH TRAINING

TRAINING TYPE	TARGETED MUSCLE GROUP		SETS					
-----	-----		1	2	3	4	5	6
		REPS						
		WGT						
		REPS						
		WGT						
		REPS						
		WGT						
		REPS						
		WGT						
		REPS						
		WGT						
		REPS						
		WGT						
		REPS						
		WGT						

REFLECTION OF THE DAY

DATE/DAY:		M	T	W	T	F	S	S
START TIME:		FINISH TIME:						

CARDIO TRAINING

TRAINING TYPE	TARGETED TIME /DISTANCE	ACTUAL TIME /DISTANCE	CALORIES BURNED

STRENGTH TRAINING

TRAINING TYPE	TARGETED MUSCLE GROUP		1	2	3	4	5	6
-----	-----							
		REPS						
		WGT						
		REPS						
		WGT						
		REPS						
		WGT						
		REPS						
		WGT						
		REPS						
		WGT						
		REPS						
		WGT						
		REPS						
		WGT						

REFLECTION OF THE DAY

DATE/DAY:			M	T	W	T	F	S	S
START TIME:		FINISH TIME:							

CARDIO TRAINING

TRAINING TYPE	TARGETED TIME /DISTANCE	ACTUAL TIME /DISTANCE	CALORIES BURNED

STRENGTH TRAINING

TRAINING TYPE	TARGETED MUSCLE GROUP		SETS					
-----	-----		**1**	**2**	**3**	**4**	**5**	**6**
		REPS						
		WGT						
		REPS						
		WGT						
		REPS						
		WGT						
		REPS						
		WGT						
		REPS						
		WGT						
		REPS						
		WGT						
		REPS						
		WGT						

REFLECTION OF THE DAY

DATE/DAY:			M	T	W	T	F	S	S
START TIME:		FINISH TIME:							

CARDIO TRAINING

TRAINING TYPE	TARGETED TIME /DISTANCE	ACTUAL TIME /DISTANCE	CALORIES BURNED

STRENGTH TRAINING

TRAINING TYPE	TARGETED MUSCLE GROUP	SETS		1	2	3	4	5	6
-----	-----								
		REPS							
		WGT							
		REPS							
		WGT							
		REPS							
		WGT							
		REPS							
		WGT							
		REPS							
		WGT							
		REPS							
		WGT							
		REPS							
		WGT							

REFLECTION OF THE DAY

| DATE/DAY: | | | M | T | W | T | F | S | S |
| START TIME: | | FINISH TIME: | | | | | | | |

CARDIO TRAINING

TRAINING TYPE	TARGETED TIME /DISTANCE	ACTUAL TIME /DISTANCE	CALORIES BURNED

STRENGTH TRAINING

TRAINING TYPE	TARGETED MUSCLE GROUP		SETS					
-----	-----		**1**	**2**	**3**	**4**	**5**	**6**
		REPS						
		WGT						
		REPS						
		WGT						
		REPS						
		WGT						
		REPS						
		WGT						
		REPS						
		WGT						
		REPS						
		WGT						
		REPS						
		WGT						

REFLECTION OF THE DAY

DATE/DAY:			M	T	W	T	F	S	S
START TIME:		FINISH TIME:							

CARDIO TRAINING

TRAINING TYPE	TARGETED TIME /DISTANCE	ACTUAL TIME /DISTANCE	CALORIES BURNED

STRENGTH TRAINING

TRAINING TYPE	TARGETED MUSCLE GROUP	SETS						
-----	-----		1	2	3	4	5	6
		REPS						
		WGT						
		REPS						
		WGT						
		REPS						
		WGT						
		REPS						
		WGT						
		REPS						
		WGT						
		REPS						
		WGT						
		REPS						
		WGT						

REFLECTION OF THE DAY

<table>
<tr><td colspan="2">DATE/DAY:</td><td>M</td><td>T</td><td>W</td><td>T</td><td>F</td><td>S</td><td>S</td></tr>
<tr><td>START TIME:</td><td colspan="2">FINISH TIME:</td><td colspan="5"></td></tr>
</table>

CARDIO TRAINING

TRAINING TYPE	TARGETED TIME /DISTANCE	ACTUAL TIME /DISTANCE	CALORIES BURNED

STRENGTH TRAINING

TRAINING TYPE	TARGETED MUSCLE GROUP	SETS		1	2	3	4	5	6
-----	-----								
		REPS							
		WGT							
		REPS							
		WGT							
		REPS							
		WGT							
		REPS							
		WGT							
		REPS							
		WGT							
		REPS							
		WGT							
		REPS							
		WGT							

REFLECTION OF THE DAY

DATE/DAY:			M	T	W	T	F	S	S
START TIME:		FINISH TIME:							

CARDIO TRAINING

TRAINING TYPE	TARGETED TIME /DISTANCE	ACTUAL TIME /DISTANCE	CALORIES BURNED

STRENGTH TRAINING

TRAINING TYPE	TARGETED MUSCLE GROUP		SETS					
-----	-----		**1**	**2**	**3**	**4**	**5**	**6**
		REPS						
		WGT						
		REPS						
		WGT						
		REPS						
		WGT						
		REPS						
		WGT						
		REPS						
		WGT						
		REPS						
		WGT						
		REPS						
		WGT						

REFLECTION OF THE DAY

DATE/DAY:		M	T	W	T	F	S	S
START TIME:		FINISH TIME:						

CARDIO TRAINING

TRAINING TYPE	TARGETED TIME /DISTANCE	ACTUAL TIME /DISTANCE	CALORIES BURNED

STRENGTH TRAINING

TRAINING TYPE	TARGETED MUSCLE GROUP		SETS					
-----	-----		1	2	3	4	5	6
		REPS						
		WGT						
		REPS						
		WGT						
		REPS						
		WGT						
		REPS						
		WGT						
		REPS						
		WGT						
		REPS						
		WGT						
		REPS						
		WGT						

REFLECTION OF THE DAY

<table>
<tr><td>DATE/DAY:</td><td></td><td colspan="2">M</td><td>T</td><td>W</td><td>T</td><td>F</td><td>S</td><td>S</td></tr>
<tr><td>START TIME:</td><td></td><td>FINISH TIME:</td><td></td><td></td><td></td><td></td><td></td><td></td><td></td></tr>
</table>

CARDIO TRAINING

TRAINING TYPE	TARGETED TIME /DISTANCE	ACTUAL TIME /DISTANCE	CALORIES BURNED

STRENGTH TRAINING

TRAINING TYPE	TARGETED MUSCLE GROUP	SETS						
-----	-----		**1**	**2**	**3**	**4**	**5**	**6**
		REPS						
		WGT						
		REPS						
		WGT						
		REPS						
		WGT						
		REPS						
		WGT						
		REPS						
		WGT						
		REPS						
		WGT						
		REPS						
		WGT						

REFLECTION OF THE DAY

DATE/DAY:			M	T	W	T	F	S	S
START TIME:		FINISH TIME:							

CARDIO TRAINING

TRAINING TYPE	TARGETED TIME /DISTANCE	ACTUAL TIME /DISTANCE	CALORIES BURNED

STRENGTH TRAINING

TRAINING TYPE	TARGETED MUSCLE GROUP		SETS					
------	------		1	2	3	4	5	6
		REPS						
		WGT						
		REPS						
		WGT						
		REPS						
		WGT						
		REPS						
		WGT						
		REPS						
		WGT						
		REPS						
		WGT						
		REPS						
		WGT						

REFLECTION OF THE DAY

DATE/DAY:				M	T	W	T	F	S	S
START TIME:		FINISH TIME:								

CARDIO TRAINING

TRAINING TYPE	TARGETED TIME /DISTANCE	ACTUAL TIME /DISTANCE	CALORIES BURNED

STRENGTH TRAINING

TRAINING TYPE	TARGETED MUSCLE GROUP		SETS					
-----	-----		1	2	3	4	5	6
		REPS						
		WGT						
		REPS						
		WGT						
		REPS						
		WGT						
		REPS						
		WGT						
		REPS						
		WGT						
		REPS						
		WGT						
		REPS						
		WGT						

REFLECTION OF THE DAY

<table>
<tr><td>DATE/DAY:</td><td></td><td colspan="2"></td><td>M</td><td>T</td><td>W</td><td>T</td><td>F</td><td>S</td><td>S</td></tr>
<tr><td>START TIME:</td><td></td><td>FINISH TIME:</td><td></td><td colspan="7"></td></tr>
</table>

CARDIO TRAINING

TRAINING TYPE	TARGETED TIME /DISTANCE	ACTUAL TIME /DISTANCE	CALORIES BURNED

STRENGTH TRAINING

TRAINING TYPE	TARGETED MUSCLE GROUP		SETS					
-----	-----		**1**	**2**	**3**	**4**	**5**	**6**
		REPS						
		WGT						
		REPS						
		WGT						
		REPS						
		WGT						
		REPS						
		WGT						
		REPS						
		WGT						
		REPS						
		WGT						
		REPS						
		WGT						

REFLECTION OF THE DAY

DATE/DAY:			M	T	W	T	F	S	S
START TIME:		FINISH TIME:							

CARDIO TRAINING

TRAINING TYPE	TARGETED TIME /DISTANCE	ACTUAL TIME /DISTANCE	CALORIES BURNED

STRENGTH TRAINING

TRAINING TYPE	TARGETED MUSCLE GROUP	SETS							
-----	-----		1	2	3	4	5	6	
		REPS							
		WGT							
		REPS							
		WGT							
		REPS							
		WGT							
		REPS							
		WGT							
		REPS							
		WGT							
		REPS							
		WGT							
		REPS							
		WGT							

REFLECTION OF THE DAY

DATE/DAY:				M	T	W	T	F	S	S
START TIME:		FINISH TIME:								

CARDIO TRAINING

TRAINING TYPE	TARGETED TIME /DISTANCE	ACTUAL TIME /DISTANCE	CALORIES BURNED

STRENGTH TRAINING

TRAINING TYPE	TARGETED MUSCLE GROUP		SETS					
-----	-----		1	2	3	4	5	6
		REPS						
		WGT						
		REPS						
		WGT						
		REPS						
		WGT						
		REPS						
		WGT						
		REPS						
		WGT						
		REPS						
		WGT						
		REPS						
		WGT						

REFLECTION OF THE DAY

DATE/DAY:			M	T	W	T	F	S	S
START TIME:		FINISH TIME:							

CARDIO TRAINING

TRAINING TYPE	TARGETED TIME /DISTANCE	ACTUAL TIME /DISTANCE	CALORIES BURNED

STRENGTH TRAINING

TRAINING TYPE	TARGETED MUSCLE GROUP		SETS					
-----	-----		**1**	**2**	**3**	**4**	**5**	**6**
		REPS						
		WGT						
		REPS						
		WGT						
		REPS						
		WGT						
		REPS						
		WGT						
		REPS						
		WGT						
		REPS						
		WGT						
		REPS						
		WGT						

REFLECTION OF THE DAY

DATE/DAY:		M	T	W	T	F	S	S
START TIME:		FINISH TIME:						

CARDIO TRAINING

TRAINING TYPE	TARGETED TIME /DISTANCE	ACTUAL TIME /DISTANCE	CALORIES BURNED

STRENGTH TRAINING

TRAINING TYPE	TARGETED MUSCLE GROUP	SETS		1	2	3	4	5	6
-----	-----								
		REPS							
		WGT							
		REPS							
		WGT							
		REPS							
		WGT							
		REPS							
		WGT							
		REPS							
		WGT							
		REPS							
		WGT							
		REPS							
		WGT							

REFLECTION OF THE DAY

DATE/DAY:			M	T	W	T	F	S	S
START TIME:		FINISH TIME:							

CARDIO TRAINING

TRAINING TYPE	TARGETED TIME /DISTANCE	ACTUAL TIME /DISTANCE	CALORIES BURNED

STRENGTH TRAINING

TRAINING TYPE	TARGETED MUSCLE GROUP	SETS						
-----	-----		1	2	3	4	5	6
		REPS						
		WGT						
		REPS						
		WGT						
		REPS						
		WGT						
		REPS						
		WGT						
		REPS						
		WGT						
		REPS						
		WGT						
		REPS						
		WGT						

REFLECTION OF THE DAY

<table>
<tr><td>DATE/DAY:</td><td colspan="2"></td><td>M</td><td>T</td><td>W</td><td>T</td><td>F</td><td>S</td><td>S</td></tr>
<tr><td>START TIME:</td><td></td><td>FINISH TIME:</td><td colspan="7"></td></tr>
</table>

CARDIO TRAINING

TRAINING TYPE	TARGETED TIME /DISTANCE	ACTUAL TIME /DISTANCE	CALORIES BURNED

STRENGTH TRAINING

TRAINING TYPE	TARGETED MUSCLE GROUP		SETS					
-----	-----		**1**	**2**	**3**	**4**	**5**	**6**
		REPS						
		WGT						
		REPS						
		WGT						
		REPS						
		WGT						
		REPS						
		WGT						
		REPS						
		WGT						
		REPS						
		WGT						
		REPS						
		WGT						

REFLECTION OF THE DAY

DATE/DAY:				M	T	W	T	F	S	S
START TIME:		FINISH TIME:								

CARDIO TRAINING

TRAINING TYPE	TARGETED TIME /DISTANCE	ACTUAL TIME /DISTANCE	CALORIES BURNED

STRENGTH TRAINING

TRAINING TYPE	TARGETED MUSCLE GROUP	SETS		1	2	3	4	5	6
-----	-----								
		REPS							
		WGT							
		REPS							
		WGT							
		REPS							
		WGT							
		REPS							
		WGT							
		REPS							
		WGT							
		REPS							
		WGT							
		REPS							
		WGT							

REFLECTION OF THE DAY

<table>
<tr><td>DATE/DAY:</td><td></td><td colspan="7">M | T | W | T | F | S | S</td></tr>
<tr><td>START TIME:</td><td></td><td>FINISH TIME:</td><td></td></tr>
</table>

DATE/DAY:			M	T	W	T	F	S	S
START TIME:		FINISH TIME:							

CARDIO TRAINING

TRAINING TYPE	TARGETED TIME /DISTANCE	ACTUAL TIME /DISTANCE	CALORIES BURNED

STRENGTH TRAINING

TRAINING TYPE	TARGETED MUSCLE GROUP	SETS		1	2	3	4	5	6
-----	-----								
		REPS							
		WGT							
		REPS							
		WGT							
		REPS							
		WGT							
		REPS							
		WGT							
		REPS							
		WGT							
		REPS							
		WGT							
		REPS							
		WGT							

REFLECTION OF THE DAY

DATE/DAY:				M	T	W	T	F	S	S
START TIME:		FINISH TIME:								

CARDIO TRAINING

TRAINING TYPE	TARGETED TIME /DISTANCE	ACTUAL TIME /DISTANCE	CALORIES BURNED

STRENGTH TRAINING

TRAINING TYPE	TARGETED MUSCLE GROUP		SETS					
-----	-----		1	2	3	4	5	6
		REPS						
		WGT						
		REPS						
		WGT						
		REPS						
		WGT						
		REPS						
		WGT						
		REPS						
		WGT						
		REPS						
		WGT						
		REPS						
		WGT						

REFLECTION OF THE DAY

| DATE/DAY: | | | M | T | W | T | F | S | S |
| START TIME: | | FINISH TIME: | | | | | | | |

CARDIO TRAINING

TRAINING TYPE	TARGETED TIME /DISTANCE	ACTUAL TIME /DISTANCE	CALORIES BURNED

STRENGTH TRAINING

TRAINING TYPE	TARGETED MUSCLE GROUP	SETS						
-----	-----		**1**	**2**	**3**	**4**	**5**	**6**
		REPS						
		WGT						
		REPS						
		WGT						
		REPS						
		WGT						
		REPS						
		WGT						
		REPS						
		WGT						
		REPS						
		WGT						
		REPS						
		WGT						

REFLECTION OF THE DAY

DATE/DAY:				M	T	W	T	F	S	S
START TIME:		FINISH TIME:								

CARDIO TRAINING

TRAINING TYPE	TARGETED TIME /DISTANCE	ACTUAL TIME /DISTANCE	CALORIES BURNED

STRENGTH TRAINING

TRAINING TYPE	TARGETED MUSCLE GROUP		SETS					
-----	-----		**1**	**2**	**3**	**4**	**5**	**6**
		REPS						
		WGT						
		REPS						
		WGT						
		REPS						
		WGT						
		REPS						
		WGT						
		REPS						
		WGT						
		REPS						
		WGT						
		REPS						
		WGT						

REFLECTION OF THE DAY

DATE/DAY:		M	T	W	T	F	S	S
START TIME:		FINISH TIME:						

CARDIO TRAINING

TRAINING TYPE	TARGETED TIME /DISTANCE	ACTUAL TIME /DISTANCE	CALORIES BURNED

STRENGTH TRAINING

TRAINING TYPE	TARGETED MUSCLE GROUP		SETS					
-----	-----		1	2	3	4	5	6
		REPS						
		WGT						
		REPS						
		WGT						
		REPS						
		WGT						
		REPS						
		WGT						
		REPS						
		WGT						
		REPS						
		WGT						
		REPS						
		WGT						

REFLECTION OF THE DAY

<table>
<tr><td>DATE/DAY:</td><td></td><td colspan="2"></td><td>M</td><td>T</td><td>W</td><td>T</td><td>F</td><td>S</td><td>S</td></tr>
<tr><td>START TIME:</td><td></td><td>FINISH TIME:</td><td colspan="8"></td></tr>
</table>

CARDIO TRAINING

TRAINING TYPE	TARGETED TIME /DISTANCE	ACTUAL TIME /DISTANCE	CALORIES BURNED

STRENGTH TRAINING

TRAINING TYPE	TARGETED MUSCLE GROUP	SETS		1	2	3	4	5	6
-----	-----			<u>1</u>	<u>2</u>	<u>3</u>	<u>4</u>	<u>5</u>	<u>6</u>
		REPS							
		WGT							
		REPS							
		WGT							
		REPS							
		WGT							
		REPS							
		WGT							
		REPS							
		WGT							
		REPS							
		WGT							
		REPS							
		WGT							

REFLECTION OF THE DAY

<table>
<tr><td>DATE/DAY:</td><td></td><td>M</td><td>T</td><td>W</td><td>T</td><td>F</td><td>S</td><td>S</td></tr>
<tr><td>START TIME:</td><td></td><td colspan="2">FINISH TIME:</td><td colspan="5"></td></tr>
</table>

CARDIO TRAINING

TRAINING TYPE	TARGETED TIME /DISTANCE	ACTUAL TIME /DISTANCE	CALORIES BURNED

STRENGTH TRAINING

TRAINING TYPE	TARGETED MUSCLE GROUP	SETS		1	2	3	4	5	6
-----	-----								
		REPS							
		WGT							
		REPS							
		WGT							
		REPS							
		WGT							
		REPS							
		WGT							
		REPS							
		WGT							
		REPS							
		WGT							
		REPS							
		WGT							

REFLECTION OF THE DAY

DATE/DAY:			M	T	W	T	F	S	S
START TIME:		FINISH TIME:							

CARDIO TRAINING

TRAINING TYPE	TARGETED TIME /DISTANCE	ACTUAL TIME /DISTANCE	CALORIES BURNED

STRENGTH TRAINING

TRAINING TYPE	TARGETED MUSCLE GROUP		SETS					
-----	-----		1	2	3	4	5	6
		REPS						
		WGT						
		REPS						
		WGT						
		REPS						
		WGT						
		REPS						
		WGT						
		REPS						
		WGT						
		REPS						
		WGT						
		REPS						
		WGT						

REFLECTION OF THE DAY

DATE/DAY:			M	T	W	T	F	S	S
START TIME:		FINISH TIME:							

CARDIO TRAINING

TRAINING TYPE	TARGETED TIME /DISTANCE	ACTUAL TIME /DISTANCE	CALORIES BURNED

STRENGTH TRAINING

TRAINING TYPE	TARGETED MUSCLE GROUP		SETS					
-----	-----		**1**	**2**	**3**	**4**	**5**	**6**
		REPS						
		WGT						
		REPS						
		WGT						
		REPS						
		WGT						
		REPS						
		WGT						
		REPS						
		WGT						
		REPS						
		WGT						
		REPS						
		WGT						

REFLECTION OF THE DAY

DATE/DAY:				M	T	W	T	F	S	S
START TIME:		FINISH TIME:								

CARDIO TRAINING

TRAINING TYPE	TARGETED TIME /DISTANCE	ACTUAL TIME /DISTANCE	CALORIES BURNED

STRENGTH TRAINING

TRAINING TYPE	TARGETED MUSCLE GROUP	SETS							
-----	-----		**1**	**2**	**3**	**4**	**5**	**6**	
		REPS							
		WGT							
		REPS							
		WGT							
		REPS							
		WGT							
		REPS							
		WGT							
		REPS							
		WGT							
		REPS							
		WGT							
		REPS							
		WGT							

REFLECTION OF THE DAY

DATE/DAY:			M	T	W	T	F	S	S
START TIME:		FINISH TIME:							

CARDIO TRAINING

TRAINING TYPE	TARGETED TIME /DISTANCE	ACTUAL TIME /DISTANCE	CALORIES BURNED

STRENGTH TRAINING

TRAINING TYPE	TARGETED MUSCLE GROUP		SETS					
-----	-----		**1**	**2**	**3**	**4**	**5**	**6**
		REPS						
		WGT						
		REPS						
		WGT						
		REPS						
		WGT						
		REPS						
		WGT						
		REPS						
		WGT						
		REPS						
		WGT						
		REPS						
		WGT						

REFLECTION OF THE DAY

<table>
<tr><td>DATE/DAY:</td><td></td><td>M</td><td>T</td><td>W</td><td>T</td><td>F</td><td>S</td><td>S</td></tr>
<tr><td>START TIME:</td><td>FINISH TIME:</td><td colspan="7"></td></tr>
</table>

CARDIO TRAINING

TRAINING TYPE	TARGETED TIME /DISTANCE	ACTUAL TIME /DISTANCE	CALORIES BURNED

STRENGTH TRAINING

TRAINING TYPE	TARGETED MUSCLE GROUP	SETS	1	2	3	4	5	6
-----	-----							
		REPS						
		WGT						
		REPS						
		WGT						
		REPS						
		WGT						
		REPS						
		WGT						
		REPS						
		WGT						
		REPS						
		WGT						
		REPS						
		WGT						

REFLECTION OF THE DAY

DATE/DAY:			M	T	W	T	F	S	S
START TIME:		FINISH TIME:							

CARDIO TRAINING

TRAINING TYPE	TARGETED TIME /DISTANCE	ACTUAL TIME /DISTANCE	CALORIES BURNED

STRENGTH TRAINING

TRAINING TYPE	TARGETED MUSCLE GROUP		SETS					
-----	-----		**1**	**2**	**3**	**4**	**5**	**6**
		REPS						
		WGT						
		REPS						
		WGT						
		REPS						
		WGT						
		REPS						
		WGT						
		REPS						
		WGT						
		REPS						
		WGT						
		REPS						
		WGT						

REFLECTION OF THE DAY

<table>
<tr><td>DATE/DAY:</td><td colspan="2"></td><td>M</td><td>T</td><td>W</td><td>T</td><td>F</td><td>S</td><td>S</td></tr>
<tr><td>START TIME:</td><td></td><td>FINISH TIME:</td><td colspan="7"></td></tr>
</table>

CARDIO TRAINING

TRAINING TYPE	TARGETED TIME /DISTANCE	ACTUAL TIME /DISTANCE	CALORIES BURNED

STRENGTH TRAINING

TRAINING TYPE	TARGETED MUSCLE GROUP		SETS					
-----	-----		**1**	**2**	**3**	**4**	**5**	**6**
		REPS						
		WGT						
		REPS						
		WGT						
		REPS						
		WGT						
		REPS						
		WGT						
		REPS						
		WGT						
		REPS						
		WGT						
		REPS						
		WGT						

REFLECTION OF THE DAY

DATE/DAY:			M	T	W	T	F	S	S
START TIME:		FINISH TIME:							

CARDIO TRAINING

TRAINING TYPE	TARGETED TIME /DISTANCE	ACTUAL TIME /DISTANCE	CALORIES BURNED

STRENGTH TRAINING

TRAINING TYPE	TARGETED MUSCLE GROUP		SETS					
-----	-----		1	2	3	4	5	6
		REPS						
		WGT						
		REPS						
		WGT						
		REPS						
		WGT						
		REPS						
		WGT						
		REPS						
		WGT						
		REPS						
		WGT						
		REPS						
		WGT						

REFLECTION OF THE DAY

DATE/DAY:					M	T	W	T	F	S	S
START TIME:		FINISH TIME:									

CARDIO TRAINING

TRAINING TYPE	TARGETED TIME /DISTANCE	ACTUAL TIME /DISTANCE	CALORIES BURNED

STRENGTH TRAINING

TRAINING TYPE	TARGETED MUSCLE GROUP		SETS					
-----	-----		**1**	**2**	**3**	**4**	**5**	**6**
		REPS						
		WGT						
		REPS						
		WGT						
		REPS						
		WGT						
		REPS						
		WGT						
		REPS						
		WGT						
		REPS						
		WGT						
		REPS						
		WGT						

REFLECTION OF THE DAY

DATE/DAY:			M	T	W	T	F	S	S
START TIME:		FINISH TIME:							

CARDIO TRAINING

TRAINING TYPE	TARGETED TIME /DISTANCE	ACTUAL TIME /DISTANCE	CALORIES BURNED

STRENGTH TRAINING

TRAINING TYPE	TARGETED MUSCLE GROUP	SETS							
-----	-----		**1**	**2**	**3**	**4**	**5**	**6**	
		REPS							
		WGT							
		REPS							
		WGT							
		REPS							
		WGT							
		REPS							
		WGT							
		REPS							
		WGT							
		REPS							
		WGT							
		REPS							
		WGT							

REFLECTION OF THE DAY

DATE/DAY:			M	T	W	T	F	S	S
START TIME:		FINISH TIME:							

CARDIO TRAINING

TRAINING TYPE	TARGETED TIME /DISTANCE	ACTUAL TIME /DISTANCE	CALORIES BURNED

STRENGTH TRAINING

TRAINING TYPE	TARGETED MUSCLE GROUP	SETS						
-----	-----		**1**	**2**	**3**	**4**	**5**	**6**
		REPS						
		WGT						
		REPS						
		WGT						
		REPS						
		WGT						
		REPS						
		WGT						
		REPS						
		WGT						
		REPS						
		WGT						
		REPS						
		WGT						

REFLECTION OF THE DAY

DATE/DAY:			M	T	W	T	F	S	S
START TIME:		FINISH TIME:							

CARDIO TRAINING

TRAINING TYPE	TARGETED TIME /DISTANCE	ACTUAL TIME /DISTANCE	CALORIES BURNED

STRENGTH TRAINING

TRAINING TYPE	TARGETED MUSCLE GROUP		SETS					
-----	-----		1	2	3	4	5	6
		REPS						
		WGT						
		REPS						
		WGT						
		REPS						
		WGT						
		REPS						
		WGT						
		REPS						
		WGT						
		REPS						
		WGT						
		REPS						
		WGT						

REFLECTION OF THE DAY

DATE/DAY:			M	T	W	T	F	S	S
START TIME:		FINISH TIME:							

CARDIO TRAINING

TRAINING TYPE	TARGETED TIME /DISTANCE	ACTUAL TIME /DISTANCE	CALORIES BURNED

STRENGTH TRAINING

TRAINING TYPE	TARGETED MUSCLE GROUP		SETS					
-----	-----		**1**	**2**	**3**	**4**	**5**	**6**
		REPS						
		WGT						
		REPS						
		WGT						
		REPS						
		WGT						
		REPS						
		WGT						
		REPS						
		WGT						
		REPS						
		WGT						
		REPS						
		WGT						

REFLECTION OF THE DAY

<table>
<tr><td colspan="2">DATE/DAY:</td><td>M</td><td>T</td><td>W</td><td>T</td><td>F</td><td>S</td><td>S</td></tr>
<tr><td>START TIME:</td><td colspan="8">FINISH TIME:</td></tr>
</table>

CARDIO TRAINING

TRAINING TYPE	TARGETED TIME /DISTANCE	ACTUAL TIME /DISTANCE	CALORIES BURNED

STRENGTH TRAINING

TRAINING TYPE	TARGETED MUSCLE GROUP		SETS					
-----	-----		**1**	**2**	**3**	**4**	**5**	**6**
		REPS						
		WGT						
		REPS						
		WGT						
		REPS						
		WGT						
		REPS						
		WGT						
		REPS						
		WGT						
		REPS						
		WGT						
		REPS						
		WGT						

REFLECTION OF THE DAY

| DATE/DAY: | | | M | T | W | T | F | S | S |
| START TIME: | | FINISH TIME: | | | | | | | |

<u>CARDIO TRAINING</u>

TRAINING TYPE	TARGETED TIME /DISTANCE	ACTUAL TIME /DISTANCE	CALORIES BURNED

<u>STRENGTH TRAINING</u>

TRAINING TYPE	TARGETED MUSCLE GROUP	SETS		1	2	3	4	5	6
-----	-----			<u>1</u>	<u>2</u>	<u>3</u>	<u>4</u>	<u>5</u>	<u>6</u>
		REPS							
		WGT							
		REPS							
		WGT							
		REPS							
		WGT							
		REPS							
		WGT							
		REPS							
		WGT							
		REPS							
		WGT							
		REPS							
		WGT							

<u>REFLECTION OF THE DAY</u>

<table>
<tr><td>DATE/DAY:</td><td></td><td colspan="2">M</td><td>T</td><td>W</td><td>T</td><td>F</td><td>S</td><td>S</td></tr>
<tr><td>START TIME:</td><td></td><td>FINISH TIME:</td><td colspan="7"></td></tr>
</table>

CARDIO TRAINING

TRAINING TYPE	TARGETED TIME /DISTANCE	ACTUAL TIME /DISTANCE	CALORIES BURNED

STRENGTH TRAINING

TRAINING TYPE	TARGETED MUSCLE GROUP		SETS					
-----	-----		**1**	**2**	**3**	**4**	**5**	**6**
		REPS						
		WGT						
		REPS						
		WGT						
		REPS						
		WGT						
		REPS						
		WGT						
		REPS						
		WGT						
		REPS						
		WGT						
		REPS						
		WGT						

REFLECTION OF THE DAY

DATE/DAY:			M	T	W	T	F	S	S
START TIME:		FINISH TIME:							

CARDIO TRAINING

TRAINING TYPE	TARGETED TIME /DISTANCE	ACTUAL TIME /DISTANCE	CALORIES BURNED

STRENGTH TRAINING

TRAINING TYPE	TARGETED MUSCLE GROUP		SETS					
-----	-----		**1**	**2**	**3**	**4**	**5**	**6**
		REPS						
		WGT						
		REPS						
		WGT						
		REPS						
		WGT						
		REPS						
		WGT						
		REPS						
		WGT						
		REPS						
		WGT						
		REPS						
		WGT						

REFLECTION OF THE DAY

| DATE/DAY: | | | | M | T | W | T | F | S | S |
| START TIME: | | FINISH TIME: | | | | | | | | |

CARDIO TRAINING

TRAINING TYPE	TARGETED TIME /DISTANCE	ACTUAL TIME /DISTANCE	CALORIES BURNED

STRENGTH TRAINING

TRAINING TYPE	TARGETED MUSCLE GROUP		SETS					
------	------		1	2	3	4	5	6
		REPS						
		WGT						
		REPS						
		WGT						
		REPS						
		WGT						
		REPS						
		WGT						
		REPS						
		WGT						
		REPS						
		WGT						
		REPS						
		WGT						

REFLECTION OF THE DAY

| DATE/DAY: | | | | | M | T | W | T | F | S | S |
| START TIME: | | | FINISH TIME: | | | | | | | | |

CARDIO TRAINING

TRAINING TYPE	TARGETED TIME /DISTANCE	ACTUAL TIME /DISTANCE	CALORIES BURNED

STRENGTH TRAINING

TRAINING TYPE	TARGETED MUSCLE GROUP		SETS					
-----	-----		1	2	3	4	5	6
		REPS						
		WGT						
		REPS						
		WGT						
		REPS						
		WGT						
		REPS						
		WGT						
		REPS						
		WGT						
		REPS						
		WGT						
		REPS						
		WGT						

REFLECTION OF THE DAY

DATE/DAY:			M	T	W	T	F	S	S
START TIME:		FINISH TIME:							

CARDIO TRAINING

TRAINING TYPE	TARGETED TIME /DISTANCE	ACTUAL TIME /DISTANCE	CALORIES BURNED

STRENGTH TRAINING

TRAINING TYPE	TARGETED MUSCLE GROUP		SETS					
-----	-----		**1**	**2**	**3**	**4**	**5**	**6**
		REPS						
		WGT						
		REPS						
		WGT						
		REPS						
		WGT						
		REPS						
		WGT						
		REPS						
		WGT						
		REPS						
		WGT						
		REPS						
		WGT						

REFLECTION OF THE DAY

DATE/DAY:			M	T	W	T	F	S	S
START TIME:		FINISH TIME:							

CARDIO TRAINING

TRAINING TYPE	TARGETED TIME /DISTANCE	ACTUAL TIME /DISTANCE	CALORIES BURNED

STRENGTH TRAINING

TRAINING TYPE	TARGETED MUSCLE GROUP	SETS		1	2	3	4	5	6
-----	-----								
		REPS							
		WGT							
		REPS							
		WGT							
		REPS							
		WGT							
		REPS							
		WGT							
		REPS							
		WGT							
		REPS							
		WGT							
		REPS							
		WGT							

REFLECTION OF THE DAY

DATE/DAY:				M	T	W	T	F	S	S
START TIME:		FINISH TIME:								

CARDIO TRAINING

TRAINING TYPE	TARGETED TIME /DISTANCE	ACTUAL TIME /DISTANCE	CALORIES BURNED

STRENGTH TRAINING

TRAINING TYPE	TARGETED MUSCLE GROUP	SETS		1	2	3	4	5	6
-----	-----								
		REPS							
		WGT							
		REPS							
		WGT							
		REPS							
		WGT							
		REPS							
		WGT							
		REPS							
		WGT							
		REPS							
		WGT							
		REPS							
		WGT							

REFLECTION OF THE DAY

DATE/DAY:			M	T	W	T	F	S	S
START TIME:		FINISH TIME:							

CARDIO TRAINING

TRAINING TYPE	TARGETED TIME /DISTANCE	ACTUAL TIME /DISTANCE	CALORIES BURNED

STRENGTH TRAINING

TRAINING TYPE	TARGETED MUSCLE GROUP	SETS		1	2	3	4	5	6
-----	-----								
		REPS							
		WGT							
		REPS							
		WGT							
		REPS							
		WGT							
		REPS							
		WGT							
		REPS							
		WGT							
		REPS							
		WGT							
		REPS							
		WGT							

REFLECTION OF THE DAY

DATE/DAY:			M	T	W	T	F	S	S
START TIME:		FINISH TIME:							

CARDIO TRAINING

TRAINING TYPE	TARGETED TIME /DISTANCE	ACTUAL TIME /DISTANCE	CALORIES BURNED

STRENGTH TRAINING

TRAINING TYPE	TARGETED MUSCLE GROUP		SETS					
-----	-----		**1**	**2**	**3**	**4**	**5**	**6**
		REPS						
		WGT						
		REPS						
		WGT						
		REPS						
		WGT						
		REPS						
		WGT						
		REPS						
		WGT						
		REPS						
		WGT						
		REPS						
		WGT						

REFLECTION OF THE DAY

DATE/DAY:				M	T	W	T	F	S	S
START TIME:		FINISH TIME:								

CARDIO TRAINING

TRAINING TYPE	TARGETED TIME /DISTANCE	ACTUAL TIME /DISTANCE	CALORIES BURNED

STRENGTH TRAINING

TRAINING TYPE	TARGETED MUSCLE GROUP	SETS						
-----	-----		**1**	**2**	**3**	**4**	**5**	**6**
		REPS						
		WGT						
		REPS						
		WGT						
		REPS						
		WGT						
		REPS						
		WGT						
		REPS						
		WGT						
		REPS						
		WGT						
		REPS						
		WGT						

REFLECTION OF THE DAY

DATE/DAY:			M	T	W	T	F	S	S
START TIME:		FINISH TIME:							

CARDIO TRAINING

TRAINING TYPE	TARGETED TIME /DISTANCE	ACTUAL TIME /DISTANCE	CALORIES BURNED

STRENGTH TRAINING

TRAINING TYPE	TARGETED MUSCLE GROUP		SETS					
-----	-----		1	2	3	4	5	6
		REPS						
		WGT						
		REPS						
		WGT						
		REPS						
		WGT						
		REPS						
		WGT						
		REPS						
		WGT						
		REPS						
		WGT						
		REPS						
		WGT						

REFLECTION OF THE DAY

DATE/DAY:			M	T	W	T	F	S	S
START TIME:		FINISH TIME:							

CARDIO TRAINING

TRAINING TYPE	TARGETED TIME /DISTANCE	ACTUAL TIME /DISTANCE	CALORIES BURNED

STRENGTH TRAINING

TRAINING TYPE	TARGETED MUSCLE GROUP	SETS							
-----	-----		**1**	**2**	**3**	**4**	**5**	**6**
		REPS							
		WGT							
		REPS							
		WGT							
		REPS							
		WGT							
		REPS							
		WGT							
		REPS							
		WGT							
		REPS							
		WGT							
		REPS							
		WGT							

REFLECTION OF THE DAY

DATE/DAY:			M	T	W	T	F	S	S
START TIME:		FINISH TIME:							

CARDIO TRAINING

TRAINING TYPE	TARGETED TIME /DISTANCE	ACTUAL TIME /DISTANCE	CALORIES BURNED

STRENGTH TRAINING

TRAINING TYPE	TARGETED MUSCLE GROUP		**1**	**2**	**3**	**4**	**5**	**6**
-----	-----	SETS						
		REPS						
		WGT						
		REPS						
		WGT						
		REPS						
		WGT						
		REPS						
		WGT						
		REPS						
		WGT						
		REPS						
		WGT						
		REPS						
		WGT						

REFLECTION OF THE DAY

DATE/DAY:			M	T	W	T	F	S	S
START TIME:		FINISH TIME:							

CARDIO TRAINING

TRAINING TYPE	TARGETED TIME /DISTANCE	ACTUAL TIME /DISTANCE	CALORIES BURNED

STRENGTH TRAINING

TRAINING TYPE	TARGETED MUSCLE GROUP	SETS	1	2	3	4	5	6
-----	-----							
		REPS						
		WGT						
		REPS						
		WGT						
		REPS						
		WGT						
		REPS						
		WGT						
		REPS						
		WGT						
		REPS						
		WGT						
		REPS						
		WGT						

REFLECTION OF THE DAY

DATE/DAY:		M	T	W	T	F	S	S
START TIME:		FINISH TIME:						

CARDIO TRAINING

TRAINING TYPE	TARGETED TIME /DISTANCE	ACTUAL TIME /DISTANCE	CALORIES BURNED

STRENGTH TRAINING

TRAINING TYPE	TARGETED MUSCLE GROUP		SETS					
-----	-----		1	2	3	4	5	6
		REPS						
		WGT						
		REPS						
		WGT						
		REPS						
		WGT						
		REPS						
		WGT						
		REPS						
		WGT						
		REPS						
		WGT						
		REPS						
		WGT						

REFLECTION OF THE DAY

DATE/DAY:				M	T	W	T	F	S	S
START TIME:		FINISH TIME:								

CARDIO TRAINING

TRAINING TYPE	TARGETED TIME /DISTANCE	ACTUAL TIME /DISTANCE	CALORIES BURNED

STRENGTH TRAINING

TRAINING TYPE	TARGETED MUSCLE GROUP		SETS					
-----	-----		1	2	3	4	5	6
		REPS						
		WGT						
		REPS						
		WGT						
		REPS						
		WGT						
		REPS						
		WGT						
		REPS						
		WGT						
		REPS						
		WGT						
		REPS						
		WGT						

REFLECTION OF THE DAY

DATE/DAY:			M	T	W	T	F	S	S
START TIME:		FINISH TIME:							

CARDIO TRAINING

TRAINING TYPE	TARGETED TIME /DISTANCE	ACTUAL TIME /DISTANCE	CALORIES BURNED

STRENGTH TRAINING

TRAINING TYPE	TARGETED MUSCLE GROUP		SETS					
-----	-----		**1**	**2**	**3**	**4**	**5**	**6**
		REPS						
		WGT						
		REPS						
		WGT						
		REPS						
		WGT						
		REPS						
		WGT						
		REPS						
		WGT						
		REPS						
		WGT						
		REPS						
		WGT						

REFLECTION OF THE DAY

| DATE/DAY: | | | M | T | W | T | F | S | S |
| START TIME: | | FINISH TIME: | | | | | | | |

CARDIO TRAINING

TRAINING TYPE	TARGETED TIME /DISTANCE	ACTUAL TIME /DISTANCE	CALORIES BURNED

STRENGTH TRAINING

TRAINING TYPE	TARGETED MUSCLE GROUP		1	2	3	4	5	6
-----	-----							
		REPS						
		WGT						
		REPS						
		WGT						
		REPS						
		WGT						
		REPS						
		WGT						
		REPS						
		WGT						
		REPS						
		WGT						
		REPS						
		WGT						

REFLECTION OF THE DAY

DATE/DAY:			M	T	W	T	F	S	S
START TIME:		FINISH TIME:							

CARDIO TRAINING

TRAINING TYPE	TARGETED TIME /DISTANCE	ACTUAL TIME /DISTANCE	CALORIES BURNED

STRENGTH TRAINING

TRAINING TYPE	TARGETED MUSCLE GROUP		SETS					
-----	-----		1	2	3	4	5	6
		REPS						
		WGT						
		REPS						
		WGT						
		REPS						
		WGT						
		REPS						
		WGT						
		REPS						
		WGT						
		REPS						
		WGT						
		REPS						
		WGT						

REFLECTION OF THE DAY

<table>
<tr><td>DATE/DAY:</td><td></td><td>M</td><td>T</td><td>W</td><td>T</td><td>F</td><td>S</td><td>S</td></tr>
<tr><td>START TIME:</td><td></td><td>FINISH TIME:</td><td colspan="6"></td></tr>
</table>

CARDIO TRAINING

TRAINING TYPE	TARGETED TIME /DISTANCE	ACTUAL TIME /DISTANCE	CALORIES BURNED

STRENGTH TRAINING

TRAINING TYPE	TARGETED MUSCLE GROUP		SETS					
-----	-----		**1**	**2**	**3**	**4**	**5**	**6**
		REPS						
		WGT						
		REPS						
		WGT						
		REPS						
		WGT						
		REPS						
		WGT						
		REPS						
		WGT						
		REPS						
		WGT						
		REPS						
		WGT						

REFLECTION OF THE DAY

DATE/DAY:			M	T	W	T	F	S	S
START TIME:		FINISH TIME:							

CARDIO TRAINING

TRAINING TYPE	TARGETED TIME /DISTANCE	ACTUAL TIME /DISTANCE	CALORIES BURNED

STRENGTH TRAINING

TRAINING TYPE	TARGETED MUSCLE GROUP		SETS					
-----	-----		**1**	**2**	**3**	**4**	**5**	**6**
		REPS						
		WGT						
		REPS						
		WGT						
		REPS						
		WGT						
		REPS						
		WGT						
		REPS						
		WGT						
		REPS						
		WGT						
		REPS						
		WGT						

REFLECTION OF THE DAY

<table>
<tr><td>DATE/DAY:</td><td colspan="2"></td><td>M</td><td>T</td><td>W</td><td>T</td><td>F</td><td>S</td><td>S</td></tr>
<tr><td>START TIME:</td><td>FINISH TIME:</td><td colspan="8"></td></tr>
</table>

CARDIO TRAINING

TRAINING TYPE	TARGETED TIME /DISTANCE	ACTUAL TIME /DISTANCE	CALORIES BURNED

STRENGTH TRAINING

TRAINING TYPE	TARGETED MUSCLE GROUP	SETS		1	2	3	4	5	6
-----	-----								
		REPS							
		WGT							
		REPS							
		WGT							
		REPS							
		WGT							
		REPS							
		WGT							
		REPS							
		WGT							
		REPS							
		WGT							
		REPS							
		WGT							

REFLECTION OF THE DAY

DATE/DAY:			M	T	W	T	F	S	S
START TIME:		FINISH TIME:							

CARDIO TRAINING

TRAINING TYPE	TARGETED TIME /DISTANCE	ACTUAL TIME /DISTANCE	CALORIES BURNED

STRENGTH TRAINING

TRAINING TYPE	TARGETED MUSCLE GROUP	SETS						
-----	-----		**1**	**2**	**3**	**4**	**5**	**6**
		REPS						
		WGT						
		REPS						
		WGT						
		REPS						
		WGT						
		REPS						
		WGT						
		REPS						
		WGT						
		REPS						
		WGT						
		REPS						
		WGT						

REFLECTION OF THE DAY

| DATE/DAY: | | | M | T | W | T | F | S | S |
| START TIME: | | FINISH TIME: | | | | | | | |

CARDIO TRAINING

TRAINING TYPE	TARGETED TIME /DISTANCE	ACTUAL TIME /DISTANCE	CALORIES BURNED

STRENGTH TRAINING

TRAINING TYPE	TARGETED MUSCLE GROUP		SETS					
-----	-----		1	2	3	4	5	6
		REPS						
		WGT						
		REPS						
		WGT						
		REPS						
		WGT						
		REPS						
		WGT						
		REPS						
		WGT						
		REPS						
		WGT						
		REPS						
		WGT						

REFLECTION OF THE DAY

DATE/DAY:			M	T	W	T	F	S	S
START TIME:		FINISH TIME:							

CARDIO TRAINING

TRAINING TYPE	TARGETED TIME /DISTANCE	ACTUAL TIME /DISTANCE	CALORIES BURNED

STRENGTH TRAINING

TRAINING TYPE	TARGETED MUSCLE GROUP		SETS					
-----	-----		1	2	3	4	5	6
		REPS						
		WGT						
		REPS						
		WGT						
		REPS						
		WGT						
		REPS						
		WGT						
		REPS						
		WGT						
		REPS						
		WGT						
		REPS						
		WGT						

REFLECTION OF THE DAY

| DATE/DAY: | | | M | T | W | T | F | S | S |
| START TIME: | | FINISH TIME: | | | | | | | |

CARDIO TRAINING

TRAINING TYPE	TARGETED TIME /DISTANCE	ACTUAL TIME /DISTANCE	CALORIES BURNED

STRENGTH TRAINING

TRAINING TYPE	TARGETED MUSCLE GROUP		SETS					
-----	-----		1	2	3	4	5	6
		REPS						
		WGT						
		REPS						
		WGT						
		REPS						
		WGT						
		REPS						
		WGT						
		REPS						
		WGT						
		REPS						
		WGT						
		REPS						
		WGT						

REFLECTION OF THE DAY

DATE/DAY:			M	T	W	T	F	S	S
START TIME:		FINISH TIME:							

CARDIO TRAINING

TRAINING TYPE	TARGETED TIME /DISTANCE	ACTUAL TIME /DISTANCE	CALORIES BURNED

STRENGTH TRAINING

TRAINING TYPE	TARGETED MUSCLE GROUP		SETS					
-----	-----		**1**	**2**	**3**	**4**	**5**	**6**
		REPS						
		WGT						
		REPS						
		WGT						
		REPS						
		WGT						
		REPS						
		WGT						
		REPS						
		WGT						
		REPS						
		WGT						
		REPS						
		WGT						

REFLECTION OF THE DAY

DATE/DAY:				M	T	W	T	F	S	S
START TIME:		FINISH TIME:								

CARDIO TRAINING

TRAINING TYPE	TARGETED TIME /DISTANCE	ACTUAL TIME /DISTANCE	CALORIES BURNED

STRENGTH TRAINING

TRAINING TYPE	TARGETED MUSCLE GROUP	SETS						
-----	-----		**1**	**2**	**3**	**4**	**5**	**6**
		REPS						
		WGT						
		REPS						
		WGT						
		REPS						
		WGT						
		REPS						
		WGT						
		REPS						
		WGT						
		REPS						
		WGT						
		REPS						
		WGT						

REFLECTION OF THE DAY

DATE/DAY:		M	T	W	T	F	S	S
START TIME:		FINISH TIME:						

CARDIO TRAINING

TRAINING TYPE	TARGETED TIME /DISTANCE	ACTUAL TIME /DISTANCE	CALORIES BURNED

STRENGTH TRAINING

TRAINING TYPE	TARGETED MUSCLE GROUP		SETS					
-----	-----		**1**	**2**	**3**	**4**	**5**	**6**
		REPS						
		WGT						
		REPS						
		WGT						
		REPS						
		WGT						
		REPS						
		WGT						
		REPS						
		WGT						
		REPS						
		WGT						
		REPS						
		WGT						

REFLECTION OF THE DAY

DATE/DAY:				M	T	W	T	F	S	S
START TIME:		FINISH TIME:								

CARDIO TRAINING

TRAINING TYPE	TARGETED TIME /DISTANCE	ACTUAL TIME /DISTANCE	CALORIES BURNED

STRENGTH TRAINING

TRAINING TYPE	TARGETED MUSCLE GROUP	SETS	1	2	3	4	5	6
-----	-----							
		REPS						
		WGT						
		REPS						
		WGT						
		REPS						
		WGT						
		REPS						
		WGT						
		REPS						
		WGT						
		REPS						
		WGT						
		REPS						
		WGT						

REFLECTION OF THE DAY

DATE/DAY:				M	T	W	T	F	S	S
START TIME:		FINISH TIME:								

CARDIO TRAINING

TRAINING TYPE	TARGETED TIME /DISTANCE	ACTUAL TIME /DISTANCE	CALORIES BURNED

STRENGTH TRAINING

TRAINING TYPE	TARGETED MUSCLE GROUP	SETS		1	2	3	4	5	6
-----	-----								
		REPS							
		WGT							
		REPS							
		WGT							
		REPS							
		WGT							
		REPS							
		WGT							
		REPS							
		WGT							
		REPS							
		WGT							
		REPS							
		WGT							

REFLECTION OF THE DAY

DATE/DAY:			M	T	W	T	F	S	S
START TIME:		FINISH TIME:							

CARDIO TRAINING

TRAINING TYPE	TARGETED TIME /DISTANCE	ACTUAL TIME /DISTANCE	CALORIES BURNED

STRENGTH TRAINING

TRAINING TYPE	TARGETED MUSCLE GROUP	SETS		1	2	3	4	5	6
-----	-----								
		REPS							
		WGT							
		REPS							
		WGT							
		REPS							
		WGT							
		REPS							
		WGT							
		REPS							
		WGT							
		REPS							
		WGT							
		REPS							
		WGT							

REFLECTION OF THE DAY

www.ingramcontent.com/pod-product-compliance
Lightning Source LLC
Chambersburg PA
CBHW070746250726
48662CB00004B/1659